VASCULITIS DIET COOKBOOK

Nutrient-Rich, Anti-Inflammatory Recipes, Foods And Meal Plans For Managing Symptoms, Boosting Immunity, And Improving Overall Health – All You Need To Know

DR. AMARI VALERIE

TABLE OF CONTENTS

BONUS:

7 days meal plan recipes, ingredients, and detailed preparatory guidelines for Vasculitis

7 Desserts procedural recipes for Vasculitis and guidelines

7 Smoothies procedural recipes for Vasculitis and guidelines

DISCLAIMER

The information provided in this book, is for educational and informational purposes only and is not intended as medical advice. The content is not a substitute for professional medical advice, diagnosis, or treatment. Always seek the advice of your physician or other qualified health provider with any questions you may have regarding a medical condition. Never disregard professional medical advice or delay in seeking it because of something you have read in this book.

The dietary suggestions and recipes in this book are based on general guidelines and may not be suitable for everyone. Individual responses to foods can vary, and it is important to consult with a healthcare professional before making any significant changes to your diet.

The author and publisher of this book do not claim to cure or treat any medical condition. The information provided is based on research and personal experience and is intended to help readers make informed decisions about their diet and health.

Furthermore, I the author do not endorse any specific products, brands, treatments, or services that may be mentioned in this book. Any references to products, services, websites, or organizations are provided for informational purposes only and do not constitute an endorsement or recommendation by the author. The inclusion of such references does not imply any association, sponsorship, or affiliation between the author and the referenced entities.

The recipes and dietary suggestions in this book are designed to be safe and healthful. However, readers should use their own discretion and consult with a healthcare professional when necessary, especially if they have allergies, sensitivities, or other dietary restrictions.

By using this book, you acknowledge and agree that the author and publisher shall not be held liable for any loss or damage, including but not limited to special, incidental, consequential, or other damages, resulting from the use of the information and recipes contained in this book.

ABOUT THIS BOOK

For individuals seeking to manage vasculitis through dietary modifications, this "Vasculitis Diet Cookbook" is an indispensable resource. This book commences with a thorough examination of vasculitis, which includes a precise definition and an explanation of the different varieties. It explores the causes and risk factors of the disease by examining prevalent symptoms and diagnostic methods. This fundamental understanding emphasizes the importance of diet in the management of vasculitis, which serves as a complementary to conventional treatment options.

This book emphasizes the significance of diet in the management of vasculitis, with a particular emphasis on the advantages of anti-inflammatory foods.

The emphasis is placed on nutrient-rich foods that enhance immunity, in addition to a comprehensive list of foods to avoid. Additionally, this book addresses the importance of proper hydration and diet preparation, providing practical advice for individuals with vasculitis. This section functions as a guide for integrating dietary modifications into one's lifestyle to alleviate symptoms and enhance overall health.

Key nutrients, such as essential vitamins and minerals that mitigate inflammation, are thoroughly examined. This book delineates the sources of omega-3 fatty acids, the role of antioxidants, and the advantages of probiotics for gastrointestinal health. Protein sources are also addressed, underscoring their significance in the processes of healing and repair.

These insights are essential for comprehending the effective management of vasculitis by specific nutrients.

Transitioning to a new diet can be a difficult process; however, this book offers a comprehensive, step-by-step guide to facilitate this transition. It delves into the process of stocking your larder with the appropriate ingredients and the process of reading and comprehending food labels. Practical suggestions for dining out are included, and meal and refreshment planning is simplified. This section is especially beneficial for individuals who are new to dietary modifications, as it guarantees that they are adequately equipped to commence their journey.

This book provides advice on managing dietary changes in conjunction with medications, managing food sensitivities and allergies, and managing social situations involving food by addressing common concerns and FAQs. It underscores the significance of monitoring symptoms and the consequences of dietary modifications, and it offers responses to frequently inquired inquiries regarding the vasculitis diet.

This book also contains specific segments that explore the advantages of a specialized diet for vasculitis patients. These chapters include a list of anti-inflammatory foods and an explanation of the significance of consistency in dietary changes. It emphasizes the importance of omega-3 fatty acids, antioxidants, probiotics, and the most effective protein sources for healing, as well as essential vitamins and minerals.

Detailed inventories of anti-inflammatory fruits, vegetables, whole cereals, healthy fats, and beneficial herbs and seasonings are provided.

This cookbook provides practical application by providing steps to create a weekly meal plan, grocery purchasing advice, batch cooking and meal prepping techniques, and a variety of fast and simple anti-inflammatory recipes. To assist readers in initiating their new diet, sample meal plans for seven days are provided, which include breakfast, lunch, supper, and refreshments. Furthermore, there are numerous recipes for each meal of the day, such as breakfast beverages, lunches, dinners, munchies, and desserts.

Lastly, this book delves into lifestyle recommendations for the management of vasculitis, underscoring the significance of maintaining hydration, stress management, regular physical activity, and adequate sleep. Regular medical check-ups and progress surveillance are also recommended to guarantee a comprehensive approach to vasculitis management. This "Vasculitis Diet Cookbook" provides readers with the ability to make informed dietary decisions, thereby enabling them to take control of their health. This is achieved through its comprehensive and practical guidance.

CHAPTER ONE

Definition And Types

Vasculitis is a collection of conditions that are distinguished by the inflammation of the blood vessels, which can result in fibrosis, enlargement, weakening, or narrowing. Giant Cell Arteritis, Takayasu's Arteritis, Polyarteritis Nodosa, and Kawasaki Disease are among the numerous varieties of vasculitis, each of which affects distinct types and diameters of blood vessels.

For instance, Giant Cell Arteritis typically affects the arteries of the cranium, particularly the temples, whereas Kawasaki Disease is predominantly a condition that affects children and can affect the coronary arteries. It is essential to comprehend the specific form of vasculitis to develop effective treatment and management strategies.

Common Symptoms And Diagnosis

Frequent symptoms of vasculitis include muscle and joint pain, fatigue, weight loss, and fever. The type and location of the compromised blood vessels determine the specific symptoms. For example, Giant Cell Arteritis may induce migraines and jaw claudication, while cutaneous vasculitis may induce ulcers or rashes.

A clinical evaluation, blood tests to detect inflammation markers such as ESR and CRP, imaging studies like MRI or CT scans, and occasionally a biopsy of the afflicted tissue are all part of the typical diagnostic process.

It is imperative to diagnose the condition at an early stage to prevent complications and initiate effective treatment.

Risk Factors And Causes

The precise cause of vasculitis is frequently unknown; however, it can be precipitated by infections, medications, other conditions such as lupus, or an abnormal immune response. Additionally, genetic factors may be implicated. Age (with varying varieties affecting different age groups), a familial history of autoimmune diseases, and specific environmental exposures are all risk factors.

For instance, the use of tobacco is significantly linked to the development of Buerger's Disease. In addition to reducing the likelihood of flare-ups, comprehension of these risk factors can aid in the prevention and management of the condition by directing lifestyle modifications.

Vasculitis Management: The Role Of Diet

The diet is essential for the management of vasculitis, as it reduces inflammation and promotes overall health. Fatty fish, verdant greens, almonds, and seeds are all examples of anti-inflammatory foods that can ameliorate symptoms. It is equally crucial to refrain from consuming refined foods, excessive sugar, and trans fats. For example, the consumption of omega-3-rich foods, such as salmon or flaxseeds, can contribute to the reduction of vascular inflammation.

It is essential to maintain a balanced intake of vitamins and minerals and to stay hydrated to support the immune system and facilitate recovery. The quality of life for individuals with vasculitis can be considerably enhanced by customizing the diet to meet their specific requirements, potentially with the assistance of a dietitian.

Treatment Options Overview

To regulate immune system activity and inflammation, vasculitis is typically treated with medications. To promptly alleviate inflammation, corticosteroids such as prednisone are frequently prescribed. To prevent relapses, immunosuppressants such as methotrexate or azathioprine may be employed for long-term management.

Biologic agents, such as rituximab, are frequently employed in severe cases and target specific components of the immune system. In addition to medication, lifestyle modifications, such as consistent exercise and stress management, serve as beneficial adjuncts.

Healthcare providers must conduct routine monitoring to optimize patient outcomes by adjusting treatment plans and managing adverse effects.

Dietary Influences On Vasculitis Management

A balanced diet is essential for the management of vasculitis, as it reduces inflammation, strengthens the immune system, and prevents nutrient deficiencies. Symptom management and overall health enhancement can be achieved by incorporating a diverse selection of fruits, vegetables, lean proteins, and whole grains.

For instance, the incorporation of leafy greens, berries, and oily salmon into one's diet can offer essential nutrients and anti-inflammatory advantages that are crucial for the management of vasculitis.

The Advantages Of Anti-Inflammatory Foods

Salmon, turmeric, walnuts, and olive oil are anti-inflammatory foods that can substantially mitigate symptoms of vasculitis and reduce inflammation. These foods are abundant in antioxidants, omega-3 fatty acids, and other compounds that aid in the prevention of inflammation. For example, these advantages can be effortlessly integrated into your diet by incorporating a small quantity of hazelnuts into your morning oatmeal or drizzling olive oil over your salad.

Nutrient-Dense Foods To Enhance Immunity

Individuals with vasculitis need to consume nutrient-dense foods, such as broccoli, pistachios, bell peppers, and citrus fruits, to improve their immune systems. Antioxidants, vitamins C and E, and other essential nutrients are abundant in these foods. A diverse array of essential nutrients is guaranteed by incorporating a vibrant assortment of fruits and vegetables into your daily diet, such as a fruit salad featuring citrus and strawberries or a vegetable stir-fry featuring broccoli and bell peppers.

Foods To Avoid

Certain foods should be avoided due to their potential to exacerbate vasculitis symptoms. These consist of refined carbohydrates, processed foods, sweetened treats, and foods that are high in trans fats.

For instance, substituting saccharine cereals with whole grain alternatives and selecting fresh fruit over confectionery can result in substantial improvements. Minimizing the consumption of processed treats and fast food contributes to the preservation of good health and the reduction of inflammation.

The Significance Of Hydration

It is imperative to maintain proper hydration to effectively manage vasculitis, as it aids in the maintenance of circulation and the support of overall physiological functions.

It is recommended that you consume a minimum of eight glasses of water per day and incorporate hydrating foods, such as oranges, watermelons, and cucumbers, into your diet.

It is essential to maintain adequate hydration to effectively manage symptoms and promote overall well-being. This can be achieved by keeping a water container on hand and imbibing it throughout the day.

By assuring a balanced consumption of nutrient-rich and anti-inflammatory foods, effective meal planning can assist in the management of vasculitis.

Begin by formulating a weekly menu that encompasses a diverse selection of fruits, vegetables, lean proteins, and whole cereals. For example, consider preparing a grilled salmon entrée with steamed broccoli and quinoa, or a lunch salad with spinach, avocado, and a lemon-tahini vinaigrette.

Sticking to a diet that is conducive to vasculitis can be made more convenient and straightforward by preparing meals in advance and having healthy refreshments readily available.

CHAPTER TWO

Key Nutrients For Vasculitis

Essential Vitamins And Minerals For Mitigating Inflammation

To effectively manage vasculitis, it is crucial to incorporate anti-inflammatory vitamins and minerals into your diet, such as zinc, Vitamin D, and Vitamin E. For example, fortified dairy products and fatty fish such as salmon are sources of Vitamin D.

Nuts, seeds, and verdant green vegetables are rich in vitamin E, a potent antioxidant. Meat, crustaceans, legumes, and seeds are all sources of zinc, which is crucial for immune function. The integration of these nutrients can contribute to the reduction of inflammation and the enhancement of your overall health.

Omega-3 Fatty Acids And Their Sources

Omega-3 fatty acids are essential for the mitigation of inflammation that is associated with vasculitis. Fatty fish, including mackerel, sardines, and salmon, are sources of these advantageous lipids.

Flaxseeds, chia seeds, and walnuts are examples of plant-based sources. Add a tablespoon of ground flaxseed to your morning smoothie or sprinkle chia seeds on your yogurt for a simple addition. Consuming these sources consistently can aid in the management of inflammation and the promotion of vascular health.

Vasculitis And The Role Of Antioxidants

In vasculitis, inflammation is associated with oxidative stress, which is mitigated by antioxidants. Antioxidant-rich foods include dark chocolate, berries (such as blueberries, strawberries, and raspberries), and colorful vegetables such as spinach and bell peppers. For example, a straightforward refreshment that is high in antioxidants could be a basin of mixed berries with a scattering of dark chocolate shavings. Protecting your cells from injury and reducing inflammation can be achieved by incorporating a diverse selection of these nutrients into your diet.

Gut Health And Probiotics

A critical component of vasculitis management is the preservation of gastrointestinal health, and probiotics are a critical component of this. Probiotics, which are present in fermented foods such as kimchi, sauerkraut, kefir, and yogurt, assist in the regulation of intestinal flora and the reduction of inflammation.

For instance, you may commence your day with a basin of yogurt that is rich in probiotics, garnished with fresh fruit, and a sprinkling of honey. The integration of these nutrients into one's daily diet has the potential to improve digestive health and reduce inflammation.

Protein Sources For Healing

In vasculitis, tissue restoration and recovery are contingent upon an adequate protein intake. Chicken, poultry, and fish are all fantastic sources of lean protein. Additionally, plant-based proteins, such as quinoa, lentils, tofu, and legumes, are advantageous.

Try a quinoa salad with grilled chicken and assorted vegetables or a lentil soup with a side of whole-grain bread for a well-rounded entrée. The body's restoration processes and overall health are facilitated by ensuring a sufficient protein intake.

Commencing The Vasculitis Diet

To prevent yourself from becoming overwhelmed, the process of transitioning to a new diet involves making progressive adjustments. Begin by gradually integrating anti-inflammatory foods, including fresh fruits, vegetables, whole grains, lean proteins, and healthy lipids like olive oil and nuts.

Processed foods, carbohydrates, and red meats should be gradually diminished. For instance, substitute your typical refreshment with a scattering of almonds and replace sugary cereals with oatmeal garnished with berries. This progressive approach ensures that you receive the essential nutrients to manage vasculitis symptoms while also assisting your body in adapting.

Providing Your Pantry With The Appropriate Ingredients

It is imperative to maintain a diet that is conducive to vasculitis by ensuring that your pantry is stocked with the appropriate ingredients. Stock your shelves with a variety of legumes, including chickpeas and lentils, as well as a variety of herbs and spices, including turmeric, garlic, and ginger, for their anti-inflammatory properties.

Additionally, includes whole cereals like quinoa and brown rice. Additionally, incorporate a diverse selection of almonds, seeds, and nutritious oils, such as extra-virgin olive oil and avocado oil. For instance, substituting refined culinary oils with olive oil, which is suitable for sautéing vegetables and preparing salad condiments, is an example.

It is essential to read and comprehend food labels to prevent the consumption of ingredients that can exacerbate vasculitis symptoms. Concentrate on the nutrition facts and ingredient list, keeping an eye out for high sodium content, unhealthy lipids, and hidden carbohydrates.

For example, it is advisable to steer clear of a product that contains ingredients such as "high fructose corn syrup" or "partially hydrogenated oils." Furthermore, it is recommended that you examine the product for any artificial additives or preservatives that may cause inflammation. Rather, choose products that are made from whole, natural ingredients.

Organizing Your Snacks And Meals

Planning your meals and refreshments is crucial for maintaining compliance with your vasculitis diet and guaranteeing an adequate intake of nutrients. Begin by devising a weekly menu that incorporates a diverse array of anti-inflammatory foods, ensuring that each meal contains a mixture of complex carbohydrates, healthy lipids, and lean protein.

For instance, a typical day might consist of a breakfast of Greek yogurt with blueberries and flaxseeds, a lunch of quinoa salad with mixed greens and legumes, and a supper of grilled salmon with steamed vegetables. Keep yourself satiated between meals by prepping nutritious munchies such as carrot spears with hummus or apple slices with almond butter.

Guidance For Dining Out

Dining out while adhering to a vasculitis diet can be difficult, but it is feasible with proper preparation. Before departing, consult the restaurant's online menu to determine appropriate choices, or contact the establishment beforehand to inquire about specific dietary requirements. Select dishes that are roasted, steamed, or grilled, and request dressings and sauces on the side to regulate unhealthy lipids and added carbohydrates.

For example, instead of selecting a fried entrée, opt for a grilled poultry salad with a vinaigrette on the side. Please do not hesitate to request modifications, such as substituting fries for a side of steamed vegetables.

CHAPTER THREE

Frequently Asked Questions And Common Concerns

It is entirely normal to have queries and apprehensions when beginning a vasculitis diet. Common inquiries include the identification of foods to include and exclude, the management of symptoms through diet, and the maintenance of a balanced nutritional intake.

Furthermore, individuals frequently inquire about the efficacy of dietary modifications in conjunction with medications and the methods for navigating social situations and dining out while adhering to dietary restrictions. These concerns can be addressed and guidance can be provided throughout the process by obtaining support from dietitians or support groups and maintaining clear communication with healthcare providers.

Medications And Dietary Change Management

It is essential to coordinate dietary modifications with medications to effectively manage the symptoms of vasculitis. It is imperative to comprehend the potential interactions between specific foods and medications, such as the avoidance of citrus or the inordinate consumption of vitamin K in conjunction with specific medications.

Consulting with a healthcare provider or pharmacist can offer personalized advice on how to modify your diet to complement your medication regimen. For instance, the optimal absorption and efficacy of a medication can be guaranteed by incorporating nutrient-rich options such as whole grains, lean proteins, and vegetables when it is required to be taken with food.

Managing Food Allergies And Sensitivities

It is essential to identify and address food sensitivities and allergies to manage vasculitis symptoms and promote overall health. Maintaining a food diary can assist in the identification of potential triggers and symptoms, thereby enabling the removal of problematic foods from the diet.

Individuals with vasculitis may experience an increase in inflammation when exposed to common irritants, including dairy, gluten, and legumes.

Experimenting with alternative ingredients and recipes can assist in the development of flavorful meals that are suitable for individuals with dietary restrictions, while simultaneously reducing inflammation and discomfort.

Strategies For Navigating Social Situations And Dining Out

While adhering to a vasculitis diet can present challenges, navigating social situations and dining out can be made enjoyable and stress-free through careful planning and communication.

When dining out, it is possible to guarantee that dietary restrictions are adhered to by conducting preliminary research on menus, inquiring about ingredients and preparation methods, and requesting modifications to the dish.

Furthermore, it is possible to prevent impetuous decisions that are induced by hunger by consuming a small meal or packing munchies.

Facilitating understanding and support in social settings and alleviating anxiety can also be achieved by communicating dietary requirements with friends and family in advance.

Monitoring Dietary Effects And Symptoms

It is imperative to consistently monitor the effects of dietary changes and symptoms to optimize the management of vasculitis. Keeping a symptom diary can assist in monitoring the frequency, severity, and duration of symptoms in response to dietary modifications.

Further modifications to the diet can be guided by the identification of patterns and correlations between specific foods and symptom exacerbations. Furthermore, the monitoring of nutritional intake can guarantee that essential nutrients are consumed in sufficient quantities and that deficiencies are prevented.

Consulting with healthcare providers or dietitians can offer valuable insights and assistance in the interpretation of symptom patterns and the refinement of dietary strategies as necessary.

CHAPTER FOUR

Anti-Inflammatory Foods Should Be Incorporated

It is essential to incorporate anti-inflammatory nutrients into the management of vasculitis. These nutrients contribute to the reduction of inflammation in the body, which alleviates symptoms and enhances overall health. Examples of such foods include fatty fish such as mackerel and salmon, leafy greens like spinach and kale, fruit like blueberries and strawberries, nuts and seeds like almonds and flaxseeds, and spices like turmeric and ginger.

These foods are indispensable components of a diet that is conducive to vasculitis, as they are rich in antioxidants and compounds that mitigate inflammation.

A wide variety of fruits and vegetables provide significant anti-inflammatory benefits. Antioxidants and polyphenols are abundant in berries, including raspberries, blueberries, and strawberries, which aid in inflammation reduction. Leafy greens, including spinach, kale, and Swiss chard, are abundant in phytochemicals, minerals, and vitamins that help to reduce inflammation. Sulfur compounds, which are present in cruciferous vegetables like broccoli, cauliflower, and Brussels sprouts, have anti-inflammatory properties.

A comprehensive array of anti-inflammatory nutrients is guaranteed by incorporating a diverse selection of vibrant fruits and vegetables into one's diet.

The Advantages Of Whole Cereals

Due to their high nutrient content and fiber content, which promotes digestive health and aids in inflammation regulation, whole grains are an essential component of a vasculitis diet. Oats, quinoa, brown rice, barley, and whole wheat are all examples of whole grains.

These grains are a source of essential vitamins, minerals, and antioxidants that are beneficial for overall health. Furthermore, the fiber present in whole grains has the potential to assist in the management of vasculitis symptoms by promoting satiety and stabilizing blood sugar levels.

Utilize Nutritious Oils And Lipids.

Incorporating nutritious lipids and oils into one's diet can be beneficial for the management of vasculitis, as it can reduce inflammation and promote cardiovascular health. Choose sources of unsaturated lipids, including almonds, hazelnuts, and avocado oil. Omega-3 fatty acids, which possess potent anti-inflammatory properties, are abundant in oily fish such as salmon, trout, and sardines. These lipids are advantageous for individuals with vasculitis because they regulate the body's inflammatory response and enhance the integrity of blood vessels.

Spices And Herbal Infusions That Mitigate Inflammation

Herbal beverages and spices are exceptional additions to a vasculitis diet, as they provide both therapeutic benefits and flavor. Curcumin, the active compound in turmeric, is renowned for its potent anti-inflammatory properties. Ginger, another spice that is frequently employed in cookery and tea, contains gingerol, which exhibits comparable anti-inflammatory properties. Green tea is abundant in catechins, which are antioxidants that promote cardiovascular health and reduce inflammation. By incorporating these herbal teas and seasonings into your daily regimen, you can improve your overall well-being and increase the anti-inflammatory effects of your diet.

Foods To Avoid

Certain foods that can exacerbate inflammation must be avoided to manage the symptoms of vasculitis. These foods, such as white bread, pasta, and pastries, are processed and refined and may contain additives that elicit immune responses. However, they are devoid of essential nutrients.

Limiting the consumption of sugary foods and beverages, including sodas, chocolates, and sweetened munchies, is also recommended, as they can elevate blood sugar levels and exacerbate inflammation.

Furthermore, it is advisable to reduce the consumption of foods that are high in harmful lipids, such as fried foods and high-fat dairy products, as they have the potential to exacerbate inflammation and increase the likelihood of cardiovascular complications associated with vasculitis.

Potential Allergens and Their Effects: It is essential to identify and prevent potential allergens to manage vasculitis symptoms. In susceptible individuals, common allergens such as gluten, dairy, and legumes can elicit inflammatory responses, which can exacerbate the symptoms of vasculitis.

It is imperative to meticulously examine food labels and remain cognizant of concealed allergens in processed foods.

Maintaining a food diary can assist in the identification of specific triggers to eliminate from one's diet and the monitoring of any adverse reactions.

Tips for Eliminating Trigger Foods: Although it may be difficult, it is imperative to eliminate trigger foods from one's diet to effectively manage symptoms of vasculitis. Begin by progressively eliminating one type of food at a time, such as dairy or gluten, and observe your body's response.

Substitute triggers foods with healthier alternatives, such as almond milk in place of dairy milk or quinoa in place of wheat-based cereals. Ensure that your meals are both pleasurable and gratifying while adhering to your dietary restrictions by experimenting with new recipes and ingredients.

Processed and refined foods should be excluded from a vasculitis diet due to their elevated levels of additives, preservatives, and refined carbohydrates, which can exacerbate symptoms and induce inflammation.

Alternatively, choose unprocessed, whole foods such as fruits, vegetables, lean proteins, and whole cereals, which are rich in essential nutrients and promote overall health. Substitute white bread and pasta with whole grain alternatives, and opt for fresh or frozen fruits and vegetables over canned alternatives, which may contain added carbohydrates or sodium.

Sugary Foods and Beverages: To prevent inflammation and blood sugar increases, it is recommended that sugary foods and beverages be restricted in a vasculitis diet.

Sugary cereals, chocolates, confectionary, and sweetened beverages such as soda and fruit juice should be avoided, as they can exacerbate inflammation and elevate the likelihood of complications associated with vasculitis. Alternatively, you may satiate your sweet appetite by indulging in naturally sweet fruits such as berries or a small piece of dark chocolate, which offer antioxidants and fiber without the addition of sugar.

To maintain your overall health and remain hydrated, choose unsweetened alternatives to sugary beverages, herbal tea, or water.

Meal Planning And Preparation

A weekly menu plan for a vasculitis diet necessitates the consideration of a multitude of factors, including personal preferences, food sensitivities, and nutritional requirements.

Begin by delineating the meals for each day of the week, ensuring that they contain a healthy balance of lean proteins, whole cereals, fruits, vegetables, and healthy lipids.

Support overall health by incorporating recipes that emphasize anti-inflammatory ingredients. Ensure that you are consuming a variety of nutrients by aiming for colorful and diverse meals and taking into account any dietary restrictions. Create a purchasing list that is tailored to your meal plan to simplify the grocery shopping process and mitigate the urge to purchase unhealthy items.

To ensure that you have nutritious meals readily available and to save time during hectic weekdays, consider using batch cooking and meal preparation techniques.

Strategies For Grocery Shopping With A Vasculitis Diet

Focus on purchasing fresh, whole foods when grocery shopping for a vasculitis diet, while avoiding processed and packaged items that may contain additives or preservatives. When feasible, prioritize organic alternatives to reduce exposure to pesticides and other hazardous chemicals. Attempt to browse the perimeter of the grocery store, which is where fresh produce, lean proteins, and whole cereals are typically found.

Thoroughly examine labels to identify potential allergens, artificial ingredients, and added carbohydrates. Stock up on pantry staples, including nuts, seeds, quinoa, lentils, and legumes, to incorporate into meals and munchies.

To obtain seasonal, locally grown produce, contemplate purchasing at local farmers' markets or enrolling in a community-supported agriculture (CSA) program.

Techniques For Batch Cooking And Meal Preparation

Throughout the week, it is crucial to have a variety of healthful options available and to simplify meal preparation by utilizing batch cooking and meal preparation. Devote one or two days per week to batch cookery, which involves the preparation of large quantities of staple ingredients, including cereals, proteins, and roasted vegetables.

Divide prepared components into individual portions and store them in hermetic containers in the refrigerator or freezer. Utilize ingredients that are adaptable and can be readily integrated into a variety of dishes, such as quinoa, roasted sweet potatoes, and grilled poultry. Invest in mason jars or meal prep containers to divide meals for easy grab-and-go. To maintain the nutritional and flavorful quality of your dishes, experiment with a variety of culinary methods, including sautéing, grilling, and baking.

Anti-Inflammatory Recipes That Are Quick And Simple

The integration of simple and rapid anti-inflammatory recipes into your vasculitis diet can contribute to the body's overall health and the reduction of inflammation. Seek recipes that incorporate ingredients that are recognized for their anti-inflammatory properties, including turmeric, ginger, verdant greens, berries, and oily fish like salmon.

Prepare straightforward dishes such as a colorful quinoa salad with mixed greens and fruit, grilled salmon with roasted vegetables, or turmeric-spiced lentil broth. To enhance the flavor of your meals without resorting to excessive sodium or sugar, ensure that your pantry is well-stocked with essentials such as olive oil, vinegar, herbs, and seasonings. To ensure that meals remain engaging and pleasurable, experiment with a variety of flavor combinations and cooking methods.

Methods For Preparing Well-Balanced Meals And Snacks

To sustain energy levels and promote overall health while adhering to a vasculitis diet, it is essential to prepare adequately balanced meals and refreshments.

To guarantee sustained energy and satiety, it is recommended that each meal contain a variety of macronutrients, such as carbohydrates, proteins, and lipids. For instance, combine lean proteins like tofu or grilled chicken with a variety of colorful vegetables and whole grains like brown rice or quinoa.

To enhance cardiac health and mitigate inflammation, incorporate nutritious lipids from sources such as avocado, nuts, seeds, and olive oil. Plan for balanced munchies, such as a sprinkling of mixed almonds, hummus, and veggie spears, or Greek yogurt with berries. To prevent overeating, it is important to pay attention to portion sizes and heed to your body's appetite and fullness indicators.

CHAPTER FIVE

Meal Plans Examples

The process of developing a sample meal plan for vasculitis entails the selection of foods that are nutrient-dense and anti-inflammatory. For example, oatmeal may be garnished with almonds and berries for breakfast, which would supply antioxidants and fiber.

A quinoa salad with spinach, avocado, and chickpeas may be served for lunch, providing a source of protein and healthy fats. Omega-3 fatty acids and micronutrients may be obtained by consuming grilled salmon with roasted vegetables, such as asparagus and sweet potatoes, for dinner.

Snacks that are both nutritious and satisfying can be provided throughout the day, such as Greek yogurt with almonds and fruit or cut vegetables with hummus.

Anti-Inflammatory Meal Plan For Seven Days

A 7-day anti-inflammatory meal plan for vasculitis may consist of a variety of delicious yet straightforward preparations. The first day could commence with a green smoothie that is prepared with spinach, pineapple, and ginger. Lunch could be followed by a lentil broth, and dinner could be broiled chicken with steamed asparagus and quinoa.

Day 2 may include a kale and quinoa salad for lunch, baked halibut with roasted Brussels sprouts for dinner, and overnight oats with chia seeds and mixed cherries. To enhance overall health and reduce inflammation, a diverse array of fruits, vegetables, lean proteins, and whole grains is incorporated into each day.

Breakfast Options That Reduce Inflammation

Breakfast options that are both nutritious and delectable can be effective in minimizing inflammation in vasculitis. For instance, a breakfast bowl that includes Greek yogurt, assorted berries, and a sprinkling of ground flaxseed contains probiotics, antioxidants, and omega-3 fatty acids.

Conversely, a vegetable omelet prepared in olive oil with spinach, tomatoes, and mushrooms provides protein, vitamins, and healthful lipids. These dishes are effortless to prepare and can be tailored to accommodate individual dietary restrictions and preferences.

Ideas For On-The-Go Lunches

Lunch options for individuals with vasculitis who are constantly on the move should be both nutritious and convenient. Wraps that are both portable and satisfying are prepared with whole-grain tortillas, grilled chicken or tofu, and an abundance of vegetables.

An additional alternative is a quinoa salad that is topped with feta cheese, bell peppers, cucumber, and mixed greens and is accompanied by a lemon vinaigrette. By preparing these sandwiches in advance or utilizing leftovers, individuals with vasculitis can maintain access to nutritious meals, regardless of their hectic schedules.

Dinner Recipes That Are Simple To Prepare

Dinner recipes for vasculitis should be both flavorful and nutritious, while also being straightforward to prepare.

One illustration is a sheet pan entrée that includes salmon, broccoli, and sweet potatoes that are seasoned with olive oil and herbs before being broiled until they are tender.

A second alternative is a stir-fry that is served over brown rice or cauliflower rice and includes a variety of colorful vegetables, such as bell peppers, snap peas, and carrots, in addition to lean protein sources like tofu or shrimp. The health benefits of these recipes are maximized for individuals who are managing vasculitis, even though they require minimal exertion.

Recipes For Every Meal

Breakfast recipes: Begin your day with nutritious options, such as smoothies that are filled with antioxidant-rich fruits, protein-packed oatmeal that is garnished with berries and nuts, or avocado toast on whole-grain bread for a healthy fat infusion.

These breakfast options offer a steady supply of energy to help you begin your day without exacerbating your vasculitis symptoms.

Lunchtime recipes: Choose vibrant salads that are abundant in verdant greens, colorful vegetables, and lean proteins such as tofu or grilled chicken.

Combine it with a comforting serving of vegetable broth or a whole-grain sandwich that is brimming with nutrient-rich ingredients, such as sliced turkey, avocado, and hummus. While managing vasculitis, these lunch options provide a balanced intake of nutrients to promote overall health.

Dinner recipes: Indulge in savory main courses such as grilled salmon with quinoa and roasted vegetables or a hearty vegetarian chili that is filled with legumes and seasonings.

For a nutritious and satisfying meal that promotes inflammation reduction and supports vasculitis management, serve these mains with sides such as whole-grain pilaf, roasted sweet potatoes, or steamed greens.

Snack recipes: Maintain your energy levels throughout the day by consuming nutritious munchies, such as Greek yogurt with honey and granola, sliced vegetables with hummus, or a handful of mixed almonds and dried fruits. While managing vasculitis symptoms, these treats offer a blend of protein, fiber, and healthy lipids to maintain a sense of nourishment and satisfaction.

Dessert recipes: Indulge in homemade fruit sorbet made with fresh berries, a small piece of dark chocolate, or a serving of baked apple slices dotted with cinnamon, all of which are guilt-free. These dessert options are suitable for individuals with vasculitis because they satiate sweet appetites while avoiding ingredients that may provoke inflammation.

CHAPTER SIX

7-Day Meal Plan Ingredients, Recipes And Detailed Preparatory Guidelines For The Vasculitis Diet

Anti-inflammatory substances should be the primary focus of a vasculitis diet, as they can assist in the management of symptoms and the promotion of overall health. The subsequent meal plan comprises recipes that prioritize fruits and vegetables, lean proteins, healthy lipids, and whole foods. Each day also includes a beverage and snack option.

THE FIRST DAY

Breakfast: Oatmeal with Blueberries

INGREDIENTS:

• One cup of rolled oats

• Two glasses of almond milk or water

• One-half cup of blueberries

• One tablespoon of chia seeds

• One teaspoon of maple syrup or honey

• 1/2 teaspoon of cinnamon

PREPARATION:

1. Bring water or almond milk to a simmer in a kettle.

2. Add grains and reduce the heat to a simmer.

3. Stir intermittently during the 5-minute cooking period.

4. Honey, cinnamon, cranberries, and chia seeds should be incorporated. Continue to cook for an additional two minutes.

5. Make plans for a hot portion.

INGREDIENTS:

- One cup of quinoa

- Two pints of water

- One can of legumes, drained and rinsed

- One avocado, minced

- Half a cup of cherry tomatoes

- 1/4 cup of finely sliced red onion

- Chopped 1/4 cup of fresh herbs

- Two tablespoons of olive oil

- The juice of one lemon

- Salt and pepper to flavor

PREPARATION:

1. Rinse the quinoa with cool water.

2. Bring water and quinoa to a simmer in a vessel.

3. Reduce the heat to low, cover, and allow the mixture to simmer for 15 minutes or until the water has been absorbed.

4. Combine cooked quinoa, legumes, avocado, tomatoes, onion, and parsley in a sizable basin.

5. Season with salt and pepper, and drizzle with olive oil and lemon juice.

6. Gently toss the ingredients to ensure they are well combined. Serve whether chilled or at room temperature.

INGREDIENTS:

• Two salmon fillets

• One bundle of asparagus, trimmed

• Two tablespoons of olive oil

• One lemon, sliced

• Two minced garlic cloves

• Salt and pepper to flavor

PREPARATION:

1. Set oven temperature to 400°F, or 200°C.

2. Arrange the salmon fillets on a baking sheet that has been lined with parchment paper.

3. The salmon should be surrounded by asparagus.

4. Drizzle olive oil over the asparagus and salmon.

5. Add lemon slices and minced garlic to the top.

6. Add salt and pepper to taste.

7. Bake for 15-20 minutes until the asparagus is tender and the salmon is fully cooked.

Snack: Almond butter on apple slices

INGREDIENTS:

• One apple, cut

• Two tablespoons of almond butter

PREPARATION:

1. Present apple slices with almond butter on the side for dipping.

INGREDIENTS:

- One cucumber

- Two stalks of celery

- One green apple

- One handful of spinach

- Juice from half of a lemon

- A one-inch slice of ginger

PREPARATION:

1. Juice all ingredients together and serve immediately.

THE SECOND DAY

INGREDIENTS:

• One cup of Greek yogurt

• 1/2 cup of assorted berries (strawberries, blueberries, raspberries)

• 2 tablespoons of a combination of nuts, including almonds, walnuts, and pecans

• One teaspoon of honey

PREPARATION:

1. Combine Greek yogurt, nuts, and berries in a bowl.

2. Apply honey to the dish and serve.

INGREDIENTS:

• One cup of drained legumes

• One diced onion

• Two carrots, diced

• Two diced celery stalks

• Three minced garlic cloves

• One can of diced tomatoes

• Four pints of vegetable broth

• 1 teaspoon of spice

• One teaspoon of paprika

• Salt and pepper to flavor

• Two tablespoons of olive oil

PREPARATION:

1. In a sizable skillet, heat olive oil over medium heat.

2. Toss in celery, carrots, and onion, and sauté until they are tender.

3. Add garlic and continue cooking for an additional minute.

4. Incorporate lentils, diced tomatoes, and vegetable broth.

5. Combine cumin, paprika, salt, and pepper.

6. Bring the mixture to a boil, then reduce the heat and allow it to simmer for 30 minutes, or until the lentils are soft.

7. Arrange for a heated serving.

INGREDIENTS:

- 2 chicken breasts, thinly sliced

- One sliced red bell pepper

- 1 green bell pepper, sliced

- One cup of broccoli florets

- 1 carrot, julienned

- Two minced garlic cloves

- Two tablespoons of olive oil

- 2 tbsp soy sauce (low sodium)

- One tablespoon of honey

- 1 tsp sesame oil

- 1 tbsp sesame seeds (optional)

PREPARATION:

1. In a large pan, heat olive oil over medium-high heat.

2. Add chicken slices and cook until browned.

3. Add garlic and continue cooking for an additional minute.

4. Add bell peppers, broccoli, and carrot. Stir-fry for 5-7 minutes.

5. In a small bowl, mix soy sauce, honey, and sesame oil.

6. Pour sauce over the stir-fry and toss to coat.

7. Cook for another 2 minutes and sprinkle with sesame seeds.

8. Arrange for a heated serving.

INGREDIENTS:

• 2 carrots, cut into sticks

• 1/4 cup hummus

PREPARATION:

1. Serve carrot sticks with hummus for dipping.

INGREDIENTS:

• Four carrots

• 2 oranges

• A one-inch slice of ginger

PREPARATION:

1. Juice all ingredients together and serve immediately.

THIRD DAY

Breakfast: Smoothie Bowl

INGREDIENTS:

• One chilled banana

• 1/2 cup of frozen assorted fruit

• One-half cup of spinach

• One-half cup of almond milk

• One tablespoon of chia seeds

• 1/4 cup of granola

PREPARATION:

1. Blend bananas, berries, spinach, and almond milk in a blender. Blend until the mixture is uniform.

2. Transfer the mixture to a vessel and garnish with granola and chia seeds.

3. Serve immediately.

Stuffed peppers with spinach and feta for lunch

INGREDIENTS:

• Two bell peppers, seeded and divided

• One cup of prepared quinoa

• 2 cups of freshly cut spinach

• Crumbled feta cheese, 1/2 cup

• One tablespoon of olive oil

• Salt and pepper to flavor

PREPARATION:

1. Turn the oven on to 375°F, or 190°C.

2. Heat olive oil in a pan over medium heat.

3. Add spinach and simmer until it is wilted.

4. Combine cooked quinoa, spinach, and feta cheese in a basin. Add salt and pepper to taste.

5. Fill the bell pepper halves with the quinoa mixture.

6. Place the loaded peppers in a baking dish and bake for 25-30 minutes, or until they are tender.

7. Make plans for a hot portion.

Dinner: Skillet of Sweet Potatoes and Turkey

INGREDIENTS:

• One pound of minced turkey

• Two sweet potatoes, diced

• One minced red scallion

• Two minced garlic cloves

• One teaspoon of paprika

• 1 teaspoon of spice

• Salt and pepper to flavor

• Two tablespoons of olive oil

PREPARATION:

1. Add olive oil to a large skillet and heat it over medium-high heat.

2. Add minced turkey and sauté until it is browned.

3. Add garlic and onion, and cook until they are tender.

4. Incorporate sweet potatoes, cumin, paprika, salt, and pepper.

5. Cover the vessel and cook for 10-15 minutes, stirring intermittently, until the sweet potatoes are tender.

6. Arrange for a heated serving.

INGREDIENTS:

• One cucumber, sliced

• 1/2 cup of guacamole

PREPARATION:

1. Serve cucumber segments with guacamole for dunking.

Apple and beetroot juice

INGREDIENTS:

• Two beetroots

• Two apples

• One carrot

• Juice from half of a lemon

PREPARATION:

1. Juice all ingredients together and serve immediately.

THE FOURTH DAY

Breakfast: Mango Chia Pudding

INGREDIENTS:

- 1/4 cup of chia seeds

- One cup of coconut milk

- One tablespoon of honey

- One mango, minced

PREPARATION:

1. In a basin, combine honey, coconut milk, and chia seeds.

2. Allow the mixture to remain in the refrigerator for a minimum of four hours or overnight.

3. Serve refrigerated and garnish with cubed mango.

Lunch: Grilled Vegetable Wrap

INGREDIENTS:

• One zucchini, sliced

• One aubergine, sliced

• One sliced red bell pepper

• One sliced yellow bell pepper

• Two tablespoons of olive oil

• Salt and pepper to flavor

• One wrap made from whole wheat

• Two tablespoons of hummus

• One fistful of fresh spinach

PREPARATION:

1. Preheat the grill to medium-high fire.

2. Apply olive oil to bell peppers, eggplant, and zucchini. Add salt and pepper to taste.

3. Grill vegetables for 4-5 minutes on each side until they are tender.

4. Spread hummus on the wrap, add grilled vegetables, and top with fresh spinach.

5. Serve the burrito by rolling it up.

Dinner: Roasted Brussels sprouts with lemon herb chicken

INGREDIENTS:

• Two chicken breasts

• One lemon, juiced and zested

• Two tablespoons of olive oil

• Two minced garlic cloves

• One teaspoon of dried oregano

• One pound of Brussels sprouts, halved

• Salt and pepper to flavor

PREPARATION:

1. Set oven temperature to 400°F, or 200°C.

2. Combine lemon juice, rind, olive oil, garlic, oregano, salt, and pepper in a basin.

3. Place the chicken breasts in a baking dish and pour half of the lemon herb mixture over them.

4. Incorporate Brussels sprouts into the dish and combine them with the remainder lemon herb mixture.

5. Bake for 25-30 minutes until the chicken is fully cooked and the Brussels sprouts are tender.

6. Arrange for a heated serving.

INGREDIENTS:

• One-half cup of Greek yogurt

• 1/2 cup of various fruit

• One tablespoon of honey

• One tablespoon of granola

PREPARATION:

1. Layer honey, Greek yogurt, and assorted berries in a glass.

2. Sprinkle granola on top and serve.

INGREDIENTS:

• One cup of pineapple slices

• One apple

• One fistful of fresh mint leaves

• Juice from half of a lemon

PREPARATION:

1. Juice all ingredients together and serve immediately.

DAY FIVE

Breakfast: Avocado Toast with Poached Egg

INGREDIENTS:

• One piece of whole-grain bread

• Mashed half of an avocado

• One egg

• One tablespoon of vinegar

• Salt and pepper to flavor

PREPARATION:

1. Toast the bread.

2. Season the toast with salt and pepper and spread the pureed avocado on it.

3. Bring water to a simmer in a saucepan and add vinegar.

4. Crack the egg into a small basin and carefully place it in the simmering water.

5. Cook for 3-4 minutes until the yolk is translucent and the white is set.

6. Serve the avocado toast with the poached egg on top.

Lunch: Corn and Black Bean Salad

INGREDIENTS:

• One can of black beans, strained and rinsed

• One cup of maize kernels

• One diced red bell pepper

• 1/4 cup of finely sliced red onion

• Chopped 1/4 cup of fresh cilantro

• Two tablespoons of olive oil

• The juice of one citrus

• Salt and pepper to flavor

PREPARATION:

1. Combine black beans, maize, bell pepper, onion, and cilantro in a sizable basin.

2. Olive oil and lime juice should be drizzled on.

3. Toss the ingredients to incorporate and season with salt and pepper.

4. Chill or serve at ambient temperature.

INGREDIENTS:

• One pound of shrimp, skinned and deveined

• One sliced red bell pepper

• One sliced yellow bell pepper

• One cup of snow peas

• Two minced garlic cloves

• Two tablespoons of olive oil

• 2 tablespoons of low-sodium soy sauce

• One tablespoon of honey

• 1 tablespoon of sesame oil

• One tablespoon of sesame seeds (optional)

PREPARATION:

1. Heat olive oil in a large pan over medium-high heat.

2. Add the shrimp and sauté until they are opaque and pink.

3. Set the shrimp aside after removing them from the pan.

4. Add garlic to the pan and continue cooking for an additional minute.

5. Stir-fry the bell peppers and snow peas for 5-7 minutes.

6. Combine sesame oil, honey, and soy sauce in a small basin.

7. Return the shrimp to the pan and pour the sauce over the stir-fry. Coat by tossing.

8. Sprinkle sesame seeds over the dish and continue cooking for an additional two minutes.

9. Arrange for a heated serving.

Snack: Dried Cranberries and Almonds

INGREDIENTS:

• 1/4 cup of pistachios

• 1/4 cup of dried cranberries

PREPARATION:

1. Combine almonds and dried cranberries, and serve.

Apple and spinach juice

INGREDIENTS:

• Two apples

• One fistful of spinach

• One-half of a cucumber

• Juice from half of a lemon

PREPARATION:

1. Juice all ingredients together and serve immediately.

SIXTH DAY

Breakfast: Omelet with Spinach and Mushrooms

INGREDIENTS:

• Two eggs

• 1/4 cup of milk

• Chopped spinach, 1/2 cup

• Sliced mushrooms, 1/4 cup

• One tablespoon of olive oil

• Salt and pepper to flavor

PREPARATION:

1. Whisk together milk and eggs in a basin.

2. Heat olive oil in a pan over medium heat.

3. Add mushrooms and sauté until they are tender.

4. Add spinach and simmer until it is wilted.

5. Pour the egg mixture into the pan and simmer until the edges begin to set.

6. Flip the omelet and continue cooking for an additional two minutes.

7. Add salt and pepper to taste and serve.

Mediterranean Chickpea Salad for Lunch

INGREDIENTS:

• One can of legumes, drained and rinsed

• One diced cucumber

• One cup of cherry tomatoes, halved

• 1/4 cup of finely sliced red onion

• Sliced Kalamata olives, 1/4 cup

• Crumbled 1/4 cup of feta cheese

• Two teaspoons of olive oil

• The juice of one lemon

• Salt and pepper to flavor

PREPARATION:

1. Chickpeas, cucumber, tomatoes, onion, olives, and feta cheese should be combined in a sizable basin.

2. Drizzle with lemon juice and olive oil.

3. Toss the ingredients to incorporate and season with salt and pepper.

4. Chill or serve at ambient temperature.

INGREDIENTS:

• One pound of thinly cut beef sirloin

• One head of broccoli, divided into florets

• Two minced garlic cloves

• Two tablespoons of olive oil

• 2 tablespoons of low-sodium soy sauce

• One tablespoon of honey

• 1 tablespoon of sesame oil

• One tablespoon of sesame seeds (optional)

PREPARATION:

1. Heat olive oil in a large pan over medium-high heat.

2. Add the beef slices and sauté until they are browned.

3. Remove the beef from the pan and set it aside.

4. Add garlic to the pan and continue cooking for an additional minute.

5. Stir-fry broccoli for 5-7 minutes.

6. Combine sesame oil, honey, and soy sauce in a small basin.

7. Return the beef to the pan and pour the sauce over the stir-fry. Coat by tossing.

8. Sprinkle sesame seeds over the dish and continue cooking for an additional two minutes.

9. Arrange for a heated serving.

INGREDIENTS:

• Two celery stalks, split into pieces

• Two tablespoons of peanut butter

PREPARATION:

1. Serve celery stalks with peanut butter for dunking.

Carrot and ginger juice: Juice

INGREDIENTS:

• Four carrots

• A one-inch slice of ginger

• One orange

PREPARATION:

1. Juice all ingredients together and serve immediately.

SEVENTH DAY

Breakfast: Almond and Banana Smoothie

INGREDIENTS:

• One banana

• One cup of almond milk

• One tablespoon of almond butter

• One tablespoon of chia seeds

• 1/2 teaspoon of cinnamon

PREPARATION:

1. In a blender, combine all ingredients and blend until the mixture is homogeneous.

2. Serve immediately.

Lunch: Salad with Roasted Beets and Goat Cheese

INGREDIENTS:

• Two beets, roasted and cut

• Two bowls of assorted greens

• Crumbled goat cheese, 1/4 cup

• 1/4 cup of roasted hazelnuts

• Two tablespoons of olive oil

• One tablespoon of balsamic vinegar

• Salt and pepper to flavor

PREPARATION:

1. Set oven temperature to 400°F, or 200°C.

2. Beets should be wrapped in foil and roasted for 45-60 minutes until they are tender. Allow to settle before slicing.

3. Combine roasted beets, goat cheese, walnuts, and assorted greens in a sizable basin.

4. Drizzle with balsamic vinegar and olive oil.

5. Toss the ingredients to incorporate and season with salt and pepper.

6. Chill or serve at ambient temperature.

Dinner: Baked Cod with Lemon and Dill

INGREDIENTS:

• Two cod fillets

• Two tablespoons of olive oil

• One lemon, sliced

• 2 tablespoons of finely minced fresh dill

• Salt and pepper to flavor

PREPARATION:

Set the oven's temperature to 375°F, or 190°C.

2. In a pan, warm up the olive oil over medium heat.

3. Top with lemon slices and drizzle with olive oil.

4. Season with salt, pepper, and fresh dill.

5. Bake the cod for 15-20 minutes or until it is fully cooked.

6. Arrange for a heated serving.

INGREDIENTS:

• Two rice cakes

• Mashed half of an avocado

• Salt and pepper to flavor

PREPARATION:

1. Apply pureed avocado to rice cakes.

2. Add salt and pepper to taste and serve.

Juice: Mint and Watermelon Juice

INGREDIENTS:

• Two cups of watermelon slices

• One fistful of fresh mint leaves

• Juice from half of a lime

PREPARATION:

1. Juice all ingredients together and serve immediately.

This meal plan offers a diverse selection of anti-inflammatory, nutrient-dense foods that can assist in the management of vasculitis symptoms and the promotion of overall health. Take pleasure in your nutritious diet!

CHAPTER SEVEN

Seven Desserts Procedural Recipes For Vasculitis Diet And Guidelines

Vasculitis necessitates a diet that promotes overall health and reduces inflammation in the blood vessels. The desserts that follow are designed to satisfy these requirements, with an emphasis on nutrient-dense options, minimal sugar, and anti-inflammatory ingredients. Here are seven dessert recipes and some guidelines to ensure that they are compatible with a vasculitis-friendly diet.

1. CHIA SEED PUDDING WITH BERRIES

INGREDIENTS:

• 1/4 cup of chia seeds

• One cup of almond milk

• 1 teaspoon of vanilla extract

• One tablespoon of maple syrup or honey

• 1/2 cup of assorted berries (strawberries, raspberries, and blueberries)

STEPS:

1. Combine almond milk, honey, vanilla extract, and chia seeds in a basin.

2. Stir thoroughly to prevent the formation of clusters.

3. Cover and refrigerate for a minimum of four hours or overnight.

4. Garnish with a mixture of berries.

Guidelines:

• Chia seeds are abundant in fiber and omega-3 fatty acids, which have the potential to alleviate inflammation.

• Antioxidants are abundant in strawberries.

INGREDIENTS:

• Two glasses of full-fat coconut milk

• 1/4 cup of maple syrup or honey

• One teaspoon of turmeric powder

• 1 teaspoon of vanilla extract

STEPS:

1. Blend all ingredients in a blender until they are completely homogeneous.

2. Pour the mixture into an ice cream maker and churn by the manufacturer's instructions.

3. Before serving, transfer the mixture to a container and chill for a minimum of two hours.

Guidelines:

• Turmeric possesses potent anti-inflammatory properties.

• Coconut milk is a source of beneficial lipids.

3. CHOCOLATE AVOCADO MOUSSE

INGREDIENTS:

• Two mature avocados

• 1/4 cup of cocoa powder

• 1/4 cup of maple syrup or honey

• 1 teaspoon of vanilla extract

STEPS:

1. Transfer the avocado interior to a blender.

2. Add vanilla extract, honey, and cocoa powder.

3. Blend until the mixture is velvety and smooth.

4. Before serving, allow the dish to cool in the refrigerator for a minimum of 30 minutes.

Guidelines:

• Avocados provide fiber and healthful lipids.

• Antioxidants are present in cocoa powder.

4. APPLES THAT HAVE BEEN BAKED WITH CINNAMON

INGREDIENTS:

• Four medium-sized apples

• Two tablespoons of honey

• One teaspoon of cinnamon

• 1/4 cup of chopped walnuts (optional)

STEPS:

1. Set the oven's temperature to 175°C/350°F.

2. Core the apples and arrange them in a casserole dish.

3. Sprinkle cinnamon and drizzle with honey.

4. Chop walnuts and place them in the center of each apple, if desired.

5. Bake the fruits for 25-30 minutes until they are soft.

Guidelines:

• Apples are a rich source of fiber and micronutrients.

• Cinnamon possesses antioxidant and anti-inflammatory properties.

5. QUINOA FRUIT SALAD

INGREDIENTS:

• One cup of prepared quinoa

• One cup of diced pineapple

• One cup of diced mango

• One cup of minced strawberries

• 2 tablespoons of freshly squeezed lime juice

• One tablespoon of honey

STEPS:

1. In a sizable basin, combine diced fruit with prepared quinoa.

2. Combine honey and lime juice in a small basin.

3. Toss the fruit and quinoa with the lime juice mixture.

4. Allow to cool for one hour before serving.

Guidelines:

• Quinoa is a source of complete protein and is high in fiber.

• Vitamins and antioxidants are present in tropical fruits.

INGREDIENTS:

• One cup of pumpkin puree

• Two cups of rolled oats

• 1/4 cup of maple syrup or honey

• One teaspoon of cinnamon

• 1/2 teaspoon of nutmeg

• 1/2 cup of raisins or dried currants

STEPS:

1. Preheat the oven to 350°F (175°C).

2. Combine pumpkin purée, grains, honey, cinnamon, and nutmeg in a bowl.

3. Incorporate raisins or dried cranberries.

4. Drop spoonfuls of the mixture onto a baking sheet.

5. Bake for 12-15 minutes until the surface is a rich golden color.

Guidelines:

• Vitamins A and C are abundant in pumpkin.

• Oats are an excellent source of fiber.

7. BLUEBERRY YOGURT PARFAIT

INGREDIENTS:

• One cup of bland Greek yogurt

• One-half cup of blueberries

• Two tablespoons of maple syrup or honey

• 1/4 cup of granola (optional)

STEPS:

1. In a glass or basin, arrange blueberries and Greek yogurt in a layer.

2. Drizzle with maple syrup or honey.

3. Granola may be sprinkled on top for an additional texture.

4. Serve immediately.

Guidelines:

• Greek yogurt is a source of probiotics and protein.

• Antioxidants and vitamins are present in blueberries.

Vasculitis-Friendly Dessert Guidelines

1. Restrict the consumption of sugar by utilizing natural sweeteners such as maple syrup or honey in moderation.

2. Select Anti-inflammatory Ingredients: Incorporate foods that are high in fiber, antioxidants, and omega-3 fatty acids.

3. Steer clear of processed foods and opt for whole, unprocessed ingredients.

4. Incorporate nutritious fats: Utilize avocados, almonds, and coconut as sources.

5. Prioritize Freshness: The vitamins and minerals contained in fresh fruits and vegetables are essential.

6. Moderate Portion Sizes: To prevent an inordinate ingestion of calories, it is important to maintain reasonable dessert portions.

7. Maintain Hydration: To promote overall health, consume an abundance of water in conjunction with desserts.

These recipes and guidelines guarantee that even individuals with vasculitis can partake in delectable, nutritious delicacies that cater to their dietary requirements.

CHAPTER EIGHT

Seven Smoothies Procedural Recipes For Vasculitis Diet And Guidelines

A diet that is abundant in anti-inflammatory foods, antioxidants, and essential nutrients can be beneficial for vascular disease, which is an inflammation of the blood vessels. Smoothies are an exceptional method for encapsulating these nutrients in a readily digestible form.

Seven smoothie concoctions have been developed to assist individuals with vasculitis. Each recipe is designed to incorporate ingredients that are recognized for their anti-inflammatory properties and general health benefits.

Vasculitis-Friendly Smoothies: A Guide

1. Utilize Fresh, Organic Ingredients: Use fresh, organic fruits and vegetables whenever feasible to

optimize nutrient intake and reduce exposure to pesticides and pollutants.

2. Concentrate on Anti-Inflammatory Foods: Berries, leafy greens, turmeric, and ginger possess potent anti-inflammatory properties and should be incorporated into one's diet consistently.

3. Refrain from consuming added sugars and instead choose natural substances such as honey or dates in moderation. Refrain from consuming refined carbohydrates, as they have the potential to exacerbate inflammation.

4. Incorporate Healthy Fats: Coconut oil, almonds, seeds, and avocados are sources of essential fatty acids that promote overall health.

5. Incorporate Protein: The addition of a handful of protein powder, Greek yogurt, or nut butter

can assist in the maintenance of muscle mass and the repair of tissues.

6. Hydrate: To guarantee sufficient hydration, utilize coconut water, almond milk, or green tea as a foundation.

7. Blending the ingredients thoroughly with a high-speed blender will result in a silky texture and facilitate the assimilation of the fibers.

Smoothie Recipes

1. BERRY ANTI-INFLAMMATORY BOOST

INGREDIENTS:

• One cup of a combination of berries, including blueberries, strawberries, and raspberries

• One cup of spinach

• One tablespoon of chia seeds

• One tablespoon of honey

• One cup of almond milk

• 1/2 teaspoon of turmeric

STEPS:

1. Thoroughly rinse the spinach and cherries.

2. Fill a blender with all of the ingredients.

3. Blend on high until the mixture is uniform.

4. Pour the beverage into a glass and savor it immediately.

2. GREEN DETOX SMOOTHIE

INGREDIENTS:

• One cup of kale

• One chopped green apple

• One-half of a cucumber

• One teaspoonful of lemon juice

• 1 tablespoon of minced ginger

• One cup of coconut water

STEPS:

1. Rinse the cucumber, apple, and kale.

2. Add all of the ingredients to a blender.

3. Blend until the mixture is uniform.

4. Chill before serving.

3. TROPICAL TURMERIC DELIGHT

INGREDIENTS:

• One cup of pineapple slices

• One banana

• One-half cup of Greek yogurt

• One tablespoon of flaxseeds

- 1/2 teaspoon of turmeric

- One cup of coconut milk

STEPS:

1. Chop the pineapple and banana.

2. Add all of the ingredients to a blender.

3. Blend until the mixture is smooth and velvety.

4. Indulge in this tropical delight immediately.

4. AVOCADO AND SPINACH POWERHOUSE

INGREDIENTS:

- One-half of an avocado

- One cup of spinach

- One-half of a banana

- One tablespoon of almond butter

- One cup of almond milk

• One teaspoon of honey

STEPS:

1. Remove the avocado interior by scooping it out.

2. Rinse the broccoli.

3. Combine all components in a blender.

4. Blend until the mixture is velvety and smooth.

5. Pour the beverage into a glass and savor it.

5. CITRUS BERRY IMMUNITY ENHANCER

INGREDIENTS:

• One orange, skinned and segmented

• One-half cup of strawberries

• One-half cup of Greek yogurt

• One tablespoon of honey

• One cup of water or coconut water

• Ice crystals (optional)

STEPS:

1. Peel and segment the orange.

2. Thoroughly rinse the blackberries.

3. Combine all components in a blender.

4. Blend until the mixture is uniform.

5. Optionally, serve promptly with ice.

6. CREAMY BLUEBERRY AND OAT SMOOTHIE

INGREDIENTS:

• One-half cup of blueberries

• One-half of a banana

• 1/4 cup of toasted oats

• One tablespoon of chia seeds

• One cup of almond milk

• 1/2 teaspoon of cinnamon

STEPS:

1. Rinse the blueberries.

2. Combine all components in a blender.

3. Blend until the mixture is velvety and smooth.

4. Indulge in a nutritious and satisfying smoothie.

7. GINGER PEACH SMOOTHIE

INGREDIENTS:

• One pitted and sliced peach

• One-half of a banana

• One tablespoon of minced ginger

• One cup of Greek yogurt

• One tablespoon of honey

• One cup of water or coconut water

STEPS:

1. Pit and divide the peach.

2. Chop and peel the banana.

3. Combine all components in a blender.

4. Blend until the mixture is uniform.

5. Allow to be served promptly for a delightful ginger seasoning.

In conclusion, by incorporating these beverages into your diet, you can obtain a plethora of nutrients and anti-inflammatory compounds that are advantageous for the management of vasculitis. It is important to consult with a healthcare professional and heed your body to customize your diet to meet your unique requirements.

CHAPTER NINE

Lifestyle Suggestions For The Management Of Vasculitis

Significant lifestyle modifications are necessary for the management of vasculitis. Initially, it is imperative to maintain a nutritious and well-balanced diet. Focus on the consumption of anti-inflammatory foods, including fruits, vegetables, whole cereals, and healthy lipids like olive oil and nuts.

Refrain from consuming refined foods, excessive sugar, and saturated fats, as they have the potential to exacerbate inflammation. Furthermore, the reduction of inflammation and the enhancement of overall health can be achieved by refraining from smoking and restricting alcohol consumption. Regular physical activity, such as swimming, walking, or yoga, can also improve circulation, and alleviate tension, and overall well-being.

The significance of consistent physical activity in the management of vasculitis cannot be overstated. Exercise enhances blood circulation, fortifies the immune system, and assists in the preservation of a healthy weight. Strive to engage in moderate-intensity exercise for a minimum of 30 minutes on most days of the week. This may encompass exercises such as swimming, cycling, or vigorous strolling.

Begin with a moderate intensity and progressively increase the duration and intensity of your workouts. Before commencing any new exercise regimen, it is crucial to consult with your healthcare provider, particularly if you have any underlying health conditions.

Stress Management Techniques It is essential to acquire effective stress management techniques, as tension can exacerbate vasculitis symptoms.

 Engage in relaxation techniques, including deep breathing exercises, meditation, or yoga, to alleviate tension and soothe the mind. Participating in pursuits or activities that you find enjoyable can also serve as a beneficial diversion and encourage relaxation. Furthermore, guarantee that you have a robust support system of friends, family, or a support group that can offer emotional support during difficult periods.

The Importance of Adequate Sleep on Health It is imperative to obtain sufficient quality sleep to effectively manage vasculitis and enhance overall health. Strive to achieve 7-9 hours of uninterrupted sleep each night.

To signal to your body that it is time to shut down, establish a relaxing bedtime routine that includes activities such as reading a book, taking a warm bath, or practicing mild stretching exercises. Ensure that your chamber is cool, dark, and silent to establish a comfortable sleep environment. Consult your healthcare provider to address any underlying issues, such as sleep apnea or insomnia, if you are experiencing sleep disturbances.

Maintaining Proper Hydration and Advice for Fluid Consumption Proper hydration is crucial for the management of vasculitis and the promotion of overall health.

To maintain proper hydration, it is recommended that you consume an adequate amount of water throughout the day, with a minimum of 8-10 glasses.

Limit your consumption of sugary and caffeinated beverages, as they can exacerbate inflammation and dehydration. If you find it difficult to consume plain water, consider infusing it with segments of fruit or seasonings to enhance its flavor.

Monitor the color of your urine; delicate yellow indicates that you are adequately hydrated, while dark yellow may indicate that you are dehydrated. Ensure that you can hydrate while on the go by carrying a reusable water container.

Conclusion

Individuals with a variety of forms of vasculitis may benefit from a vasculitis diet, which is designed to promote overall health, alleviate symptoms, and potentially reduce inflammation. While no single diet is universally recommended for all patients with vasculitis, general dietary principles can be advantageous.

A balanced diet that is abundant in anti-inflammatory foods, including fruits, vegetables, whole cereals, lean proteins, and healthy lipids like those found in nuts and salmon, is prioritized. The potential anti-inflammatory properties of foods that are abundant in omega-3 fatty acids and antioxidants are particularly encouraged.

Patients are advised to restrict or avoid foods that may exacerbate inflammation or contribute to other health issues, such as processed foods, high sugar content, and saturated fats. It is also essential to maintain a healthy weight through regular physical activity and appropriate nutrition, as obesity can exacerbate symptoms and complications.

Individualized dietary plans are frequently advised because the dietary requirements of each patient may differ depending on their specific type of vasculitis, medications, and overall health status. Consulting with healthcare professionals, such as dietitians, can assist in the development of a diet plan that is customized to meet the individual's health requirements and facilitates the management of disease.

Ultimately, a well-planned diet can be beneficial in the management of vasculitis, as it can improve the quality of life for patients and promote overall well-being.

THE END

www.ingramcontent.com/pod-product-compliance
Lightning Source LLC
Chambersburg PA
CBHW061048250726
48653CB00001B/311